Also by Daniel Stih

Healthy Living Spaces
Top 10 Hazards Affecting Your Health

Mold Money
How to Save Thousands of Dollars on Mold
Remediation and Make Sure the Mold is Gone

How to Build a Healthy Home
And Prevent the Negative Impacts on Your Health
That Can Result From Poorly Executed Green
Building Initiatives

Unplugged
How to Find and Get Rid of EMFs in Your Home

What Your Builder Should Know
Best Practices for Building a Healthy Home

DUST MONEY

How to Clean You Home and
Belongings After Mold Remediation
o You Don't Have to Throw Everything Away

DANIEL STIH
BSE, CMC, CIEC

Copyright ©2020 by Daniel Stih

All rights reserved.

ISBN: 978-0-9794685-4-4

No part of this book may be reproduced or transmitted in any form, electronic or mechanical, including photocopying, without written permission of the author, except for brief passages in a magazine or newspaper review.

Inquiries regarding requests to reprint parts should be addressed to the publisher at the address below:

Healthy Living Spaces
369 Montezuma Ave #169
Santa Fe, NM 87501

Disclaimer

Every building has a unique set of circumstances for which additional specifications or modifications of the information presented herein are required. The intent is to provide basic information that you can use to make informed decisions. The author does not assume responsibility for any actions you may take after reading this book. If you need specific recommendations, please contact Healthy Living Spaces® to make an appointment for a consultation.

Unconditional Release of Liability

You hereby release and exempt the author and Healthy Living Spaces® from any and all liability and responsibility regarding the use of any of the information contained herein.

Notice

This book is intended to supplement *Mold Money: How to Save Thousands of Dollars on Mold Remediation and Make Sure the Mold is Gone.* Whereas *Mold Money* explains how to instruct a mold remediator removing mold growing in your home or office, the book you are reading explains how to clean up the dust and settled spores that remain afterward. This book could be called *Dust Remediation.* Actual growth must be removed first. If you know or think you have mold growing, please reference *Mold Money.*

TABLE OF CONTENTS

Introduction   1
Supplies Required   15

The Cleaning Process

Cleaning or Replacing the HVAC and Ductwork   25
Cleaning the House   29
Cleaning Contents (Belongings)   43

Testing

Testing a House   49
Interpreting Laboratory Results   52
Testing Household Contents (Belongings)   54
The Environmental Relative Mold Index (ERMI)   59

Standards, Guidelines, and References   77

Introduction

If you're reading this book, you may be experiencing intense feelings of frustration and helplessness with regard to why you are not feeling better in your home after a mold remediation project was completed. If you are certain that the actual mold growth was removed, then what you are reacting to is dust in the house that contains not only mold spores but fragments of other organisms that flourished when the house was wet as well as construction debris such as drywall dust, insulation, and sawdust, the results of remediation and rebuilding activities.

    The good news is that you can make an improvement and create a healthier living space simply by cleaning the house. Just using a vacuum cleaner is not going to work. The best way to remove dust from unseen places is to use a leaf blower after you pack the contents out. This will blow an incredible amount of dust into the open, where it can be vacuumed. Add to this an air scrubber (i.e., a giant air filter), and oscillating fans to keep the dust stirred up so it can be filtered out by the air scrubber, and you will have the best possible system for cleaning a house. Using this system, you can make a house cleaner than it was when it was built. This cleaning protocol has helped people who suffer from allergies in general.

Some think the that they are not feeling better after mold remediation is because their stuff is contaminated with mold. Therefore, they think the answer is to throw their things away. This is not necessary. The issue is not that mold grew on them. Rather, it's what's in the dust that settled on them. The contents of the house simply need to be cleaned, as will be explained.

How I Know

I've had a microscope since I was twelve, when my brothers and I opened Sun Laboratorys in the utility room of our parents' home. I let milk spoil and examined what grew under the microscope. Moving forward, I got a degree in Aerospace Engineering. After eleven years working for Fortune 100 company, I quit my job, moved to a small town, and ended up working as a handyman. I had so much work that I didn't know what to do with it all. Then one day, I started to get sick and found out it was due to the hazardous stuff I was exposed to.

Introduction

I decided to find ways of testing homes and getting rid of what was making us sick. I took every class I could find on mold inspections, testing, and removal. Now, I am a Council-Certified Microbial Consultant (CMC), board-awarded by the American Council for Accredited Certification (ACAC). My certifications are accredited by the Engineering Specialties Board (CSB). I have been a consultant to the Dyson corporation, taught classes for the National Kitchen and Bath Association (NKBA), and developed courses to be taken by mold inspectors and remediators in the State of Florida, including "Minimum Standards and Practices for Florida Mold Assessors and Remediators" and "It's More Than Mold - Health Effects Associated with Mold and Water Damage." I have partnered with Los Alamos National Laboratories to study products used to treat mold. Treatment is not the answer. It won't make you feel better or get rid of mold.

Some houses have mold growth in them after a remediation company says they are finished with remediation. This happens when a mold inspector does not identify all the locations that have hidden mold to be removed by a remediator. It also happens when a mold remediator treats, but does not remove the mold that was found. But even if all the actual growth is removed where it is found, many don't consider cleaning the rest of the house or don't know how.

Dust Money

A SHORT HISTORY OF MOLD TESTING AND CLEANING

When I got started in the business, I was not taught how to clean a house after mold remediation was completed, other than to HEPA vacuum and damp-wipe the work area where mold was removed. I was not taught that I could test the house to see if the entire house needed to be cleaned. If the work area was clean, I told the homeowner that the mold was gone. I considered that if there was mold in a house for some time before it was discovered and removed, then some of the mold might have escaped from the places where it was hiding (it always does). Would not some of those particles, spores, and allergens have settled in the dust throughout the home? It had to be so.

A few mold inspectors, including myself, have tried to find ways of testing the dust in a house to look for spores in the settled dust. I collected samples of dust from surfaces and sent them to a laboratory, picking spots where lots of dust collects (the top of a door jamb is a good place). To do this, I used what is called a "tape-lift." A clear piece of tape is stuck to a surface, removed, and sent to the lab. Using a microscope, the lab examines what is stuck to the tape and identifies any mold spores on it. This is like looking for a needle in a haystack. When you find one, you can't be

Introduction

sure it is an anomaly—look hard enough and you will find one.

Advancements in the quest to use dust to test for mold in homes came along with the idea of culturing the dust. When dust is cultured, small, viable spores grow into big, fuzzy colonies, making it easier for the lab to detect them. Some testing companies have gone so far as to develop numerical guidelines on how many colonies of mold should be considered normal. At least one study has compared levels of mold in dust from large office buildings known to have mold to the mold levels in dust from other buildings. From these came numerical guidelines. Things looked hopeful. For a while.

Using studies such as this, I found it still wasn't easy to tell whether there was mold in a home. Some of the houses that I tested had mold actively growing but had dust samples suggesting that the level of mold in the dust was normal. For others, the results looked as if there had to be mold in the house. Yet after spending hundreds of dollars testing each house to find the mold, it turned out that there wasn't any. I wondered where the mold in the dust had come from. Did some of it come from outside? Of course.

I began collecting dust samples outdoors to compare to the samples I collected indoors. But that still did not answer the question of whether there was mold in a house. There are too many variables affect-

Dust Money

ing how and where dust settles.

As part of my continuing education, I attended professional conferences and seminars. In 2010, I saw a presentation on how to test for settled spores in dust by using a leaf blower to disturb the dust before collecting air samples.[1] The idea was simple, ingenious, and not without foresight. It was borrowed from the asbestos industry. After the bulk of asbestos-containing materials are removed, blowers and fans are used to disturb the dust as part of the cleaning and testing process. When the mold remediation industry was in its infancy, it borrowed the ideas of using air scrubbers and creating negative air pressures from the asbestos industry. For no good reason, it did not copy the use of fans and blowers.

The presentation was of a study in which fans were used to disturb the settled dust in a home while an air scrubber was running so that dust (settled, residual mold particles) could be filtered out of the air. A leaf blower was used to blow dust off of hard-to-reach places, such as doors jambs, lamp fixtures, ceilings, and so forth. The dust blew out into the open, where it could be vacuumed. The process of using fans and a leaf blower to clean a house turned out to be more effective than HEPA vacuuming and damp wiping alone. It's also a good way to clean the contents of the house.

This process is not recommended to test a house

Introduction

for hidden mold growth. (For this, use the WallChek® instead). Rather, this process is used to clean a house and its contents of the spores and mold particles that settle in dust and to test the effectiveness of this cleaning. This cleaning process should be used only after the areas with actual mold growth have been identified and the mold growth has been removed by a mold remediator.

Before we get into the nuts and bolts of the cleaning process, it's helpful to understand the difference between actual mold growth, mold spores, and particles that settle out in the dust.

Mold Needs Water to Grow

Mold growing in one part of the house does not mean mold grew on items in other parts of the house. Don't water it, and mold can not grow on it. Mold cannot grow on your belongings unless they get wet. In some cases, everything might have gotten wet. However, that's not usually the case, except in natural disasters when flooding occurs. If everything got wet, then maybe you should throw it all away. But unless the items got wet and mold grew on them, throwing them out is not required. The items and the house just need to be cleaned. A solution proposed by a remediator may be to fog or treat a house. That is not going to work. This is a dust remediation project.

Dust Money

THE DIFFERENCE BETWEEN GROWTH AND SETTLED SPORES

Some people say mold is everywhere. It is true that if you look hard enough, you may find a mold spore in practically any environment. Finding a mold spore, however, is different from finding MOLD GROWTH. The *ANSI/IICRC S520 Standard and Reference Guide for Professional Mold Remediation* contains definitions that differentiates mold growth from background and settled spores in the dust.

Mold growth is defined as an area where actual mold growth is currently present. Mold growth contains not only spores but hyphae (roots) and other body parts of the fungus. It is the presence of these other parts that allows a laboratory to conclude that what they are looking at is growth vs. background spores. Mold growth can be dead or alive, active or dormant, treated or not, old or new. It does not matter. Mold growth, by definition, is mold that grew on materials that got wet. Mold growth should be removed by cutting out moldy materials (e.g., drywall or rotten wood), sanding and wire-brushing wood that is not rotted, and using a vacuum, soap and water to clean up the mess, as discussed in *Mold Money*.

Cross-contamination (settled spores) is defined as spores that originated from actual growth, got into the air, and settled out in the dust onto surfaces and

Introduction

belongings. The spores that settle will not grow unless they settle onto surfaces that are wet. Spores that do not grow can be easily removed. It's as simple as spring cleaning, what is normally done to clean dust off surfaces. Cross-contamination can be thought of just as *mold*.

The best way to keep this straight is to use two words—mold growth—when intending to mean actual growth. When speaking about settled spores in the dust, use the single word *mold*.

The third category consists of background spores that blew in from outside. This is defined as a *normal fungal ecology*, a definition that I think could use some improvement. Normal is relative to a specific geographic location at a specific moment in time and can undergo random changes. The important thing to understand is that these spores are considered background spores because they came from outside, not from mold that grew in the house.

According the *ANSI/IICRC S520* standard, the goal of mold remediation should be to restore a home to a normal fungal ecology. Most mold remediation companies, however, remove the mold that grew but do not clean areas outside of the work area to remove settled spores. In essence, they do not clean the entire house or its contents. Therefore, in most cases, only the work area is restored to normal. The remainder of the house will still have settled spores.

Dust Money

Before cleaning the house and its contents as prescribed in this book, you should first contact a mold inspector and remediation company to locate and remove any mold growth present. I use the WallChek® method to locate where mold growth may be hiding, as discussed in *Mold Money*. I'm not trying to sell you two books. It's just simpler to understand the process one step at a time. Otherwise, you may find yourself overwhelmed and tempted to throw your stuff away. Stick with me. This topic is easy to understand when you break it down to the culprit at this point: dust.

Why Cleaning is Important

Mold is not the only organism that flourishes in damp conditions. Where there is moisture, they come: mold, bacteria, bugs, amoebae, you name it. Things you can't see, things you can't pronounce, things we don't want in our homes. These all have the potential to affect our health. According to the Institute of Medicine of the National Academies, while much attention is focused on mold spores, the following can be present in water-damaged buildings and can have health effects. The cleaning protocol in this book will remove these irritants as well. This is the short list:

- Cells, hyphae, mycelium fragments, filaments, and

Introduction

granules of mold.

- Mycotoxins. Some mistakenly think that mycotoxins are gases. Instead, they are solid substances that the mold secretes and slathers itself with to protect it from competing organisms. When present, mycotoxins are on all parts of the mold, including fragments.

- Spores and cells of bacteria. Actinomycetes, a type of sporulating bacteria associated with damp soil, is one example.

- Glucans (found in the cell walls of molds).

- Endotoxins (found in the cell walls of gram-negative bacteria).

- Peptidoglycans (found in the cell walls of gram-positive bacteria).

- Protozoa, such as amoebae.

- Debris from damp building materials that deteriorate into fragments and settle in the dust. Dampness can damage building materials, causing or increasing the release of chemical and non-biological particles. These particles may be saturated with enzymes that molds produce to break materials down into simple sugars they can absorb.

Dust Money

- Insects such as ants, spiders, dust mites, and roaches. Insect scales, hairs, urine, and feces.

- Allergens and irritants associated with rodents, rodent urine, and droppings. Rodents are attracted to moisture and like to build nests in the insulation.

- Things yet to be realized or studied.

Yeasts

Yeasts are a type of fungi of which there are many different species. Little is known regarding the health effects of yeast exposure. Yeasts can grow in frigid temperatures where no other types of mold will grow.

On one occasion, I tested an apartment that had flooded in the winter. The upstairs had a burst pipe, which caused the downstairs to become soaking wet and tripped the circuit breaker to the heaters. It was Christmas, and the downstairs tenant was out of town. By the time he got back, his apartment had been soaking wet for a week, and the power was still off. The temperature inside was 45°F. Testing indicated there was no amplification of mold, with the exception of significant quantities of yeasts. The heat was left off during remediation, and the tenant was able to clean his stuff and re-occupy the building after remediation.

Introduction

Protozoa

Just when you thought things couldn't get stranger, one study detected amoebae in 22% of 124 samples collected from materials with water damage. According to *Bioaerosols: Assessment and Control*, amoebae may play a role in supporting the growth and survival of Legionella, bacteria associated with illness in large commercial buildings. Amoebae feed by engulfing algae, bacteria, and smaller organisms, of which the engulfed bacteria remain alive and infectious.

Want to learn more? Check out *Adverse Health Effects Associated with Molds in the Indoor Environment* by the American College of Occupational and Environmental Medicine, October, 2002.

White Stuff That is Not Mold

Efflorescence is a white, powdery, crystalline substance found on block and concrete walls in crawlspaces, basements, and cement plaster where water has migrated through the surface. As water evaporates from the surface, it leaves salts. Although the resulting white deposits are not mold growth, they may cause symptoms. These salts become airborne and may have microscopic mold, bacteria, allergens, and other irritants attached.

Just Do It

The information in this chapter was presented to emphasize the importance of cleaning. The items listed herein are not fully inclusive of what may be present in cases of water damage. Do not try to determine the potential for your health to be affected by them based on a mold test. Mold inspectors only test for mold. It's not practical and can be expensive to test for all of them. Sometimes, it's the dust from demolition and reconstruction activities that bothers people (e.g., drywall, plaster dust, fibers, insulation, and sawdust). Don't study it. Just clean it.

---

1. "How to Determine and Successfully Clean Up Condition 2 Settled Spores - An Update," William Vaughan, PhD, Presented at the 13th Annual Indoor Air Quality Association (IAQA) meeting, Austin, TX, 2010.

Supplies Required

An Air Scrubber

An air scrubber is a fancy name for a box with a big fan inside it and a big filter on the exhaust. Inside is a blower similar to what is inside a furnace or an air conditioner. Air is pulled into the intake and passes through two pre-filters. The pre-filters capture the big dust (e.g., drywall dust) to prolong the life of the HEPA filter. After passing through a HEPA filter, the air is exhausted.

Air scrubbers are sometimes referred to as "negative air machines." This is only correct when a duct is connected to the exhaust of the scrubber and vented outside. When this is done, suction is created inside the home, resulting in a negative air pressure.

The more air scrubbers you have, the better. Ideally, one air scrubber is placed in the center of each room. Having a scrubber in each room is the most effective way of cleaning in the shortest amount of time. The only thing stopping homeowners from having lots of air scrubbers is their cost.

Dust Money

Air scrubbers are rated (and priced) based on how much air they move in cubic feet per minute (CFM). The smallest air scrubbers move 600—700 CFM and cost just under $1,000 US. Larger air scrubbers move 2,500 CFM and cost $2,000 or more. A four-bedroom house may require six or more air scrubbers to put a scrubber in every room. Most of us do not have that kind of money. Consider that when you are finished, you could do what insurance companies call salvaging the equipment: sell it on eBay for half of what you paid.

Insurance companies have been known to pay for "dust remediation" when clients report feeling sick from drywall and reconstruction dust. In one case, an insurance company paid me to buy scrubbers and fans for a project. It was not allowed for the client to be given money for the equipment. After the cleaning was finished, I sold the equipment, and the insurance company paid me the difference of what I paid to purchase and sell the air scrubbers.

If you buy an air scrubber, order one case of each type of pre-filter. There are two types of pre-filters: a coarse filter and a fine filter. Both pre-filters should be changed as they become dirty.

Buy new air scrubbers. Do not rent them. If you rent one, it should be exhausted outside, as would be done during mold remediation. HEPA means a filter is 99%, not 100%, effective. Some particles are going to

Supplies You Will Need

blow out of the machines back into the air. You don't want a rented air scrubber to exhaust inside your home. That defeats the purpose of cleaning it. If you rent an air scrubber, you should buy a box of flexible ducting and a clamp to secure the duct to the air scrubber so that the air can be exhausted outdoors.

If you can't buy an air scrubber, open the windows as you follow the cleaning process. It may help to put box fans in the windows, facing them outward and sealing around the window openings as best as possible to make a tight fit. Doing so may help to pull dusty air out of the house as you clean. It's best to purchase at least one air scrubber. It can be a small one.

Air Scrubbers / Negative Air Machines
Abatement Technologies
(800) 634-9091
www.abatement.com

Aerospace America
www.aerospaceamerica.com

Air Washer

An air washer is a fancy technical term for a leaf blower. You need a leaf blower. You can use a leaf blower you already have. Turn it on outside for a moment to clean it. A new leaf blower costs as little as $30 US.

Some use compressed air hoses instead. A com-

Dust Money

pressed air hose is not a substitute for a leaf blower. A leaf blower enables a shotgun approach: you wave it around as you walk through the house. If you use a compressed air hose, you are going to miss places. A compressed air hose can be rented from a local hardware store. A compressed air hose can be loud and heavy. A leaf blower is lighter and more portable, making it easy to walk through a house while waving it around.

Oscillating Fans

Oscillating fans are used to keep dust in the air so that dust particles can be filtered out by the air scrubbers. You can't have too many fans. Ideally, there will be several in each room and they will swivel. The swivel is important to keep the air movement dynamic and avoid stagnant zones where dust can settle. Carpet fans are OK but should not be the sole type of fan used. Carpet fans create a direct stream of air, which causes dead zones and dust to settle in the corners of rooms.

HEPA Vacuum

HEPA (high-efficiency particle arrestance) means that what goes in stays in the bag and doesn't blow out into the air. You can buy an industrial HEPA vacuum for about $1,200. I use a Nilfisk Model GM80. Miele, a

Supplies You Will Need

popular household brand, makes good HEPA vacuum cleaners. Non-HEPA Miele vacuums are known to perform as well as HEPA vacuums due to a gasket on the filter.

Personal Protective Equipment (PPE)

Wear a full-face respirator or, at a minimum, a half-face respirator and goggles. A full-face respirator provides ten times the level of protection provided by a half-face respirator. This has to do with a better seal around the face. You cannot find good ones at local hardware stores. Order one online.

The respirator should have HEPA (P100) filters. When you order cartridges, you will see filters that are a combination of organic vapor (VOC) and HEPA/P100 filters. These are two filters in one. The VOC removes odors, and the HEPA (P100) removes particles. You will only need the HEPA/P100 filters. If a house smells moldy, you shouldn't be in it, as there may still be mold growth that needs to be removed.

Order the respirator weeks in advance before you expect to start cleaning. This allows time to order another if it doesn't fit. When it arrives, put it on according to the instructions. When you are satisfied with the fit, place your hands over the filters to cover them while breathing in at the same time. It should be difficult to breathe air in. You should feel the respira-

Dust Money

tor being sucked onto your face. If instead you feel air brushing past the side of your face as it leaks though the sides, you should adjust the fit. Don't make it fit by cinching the straps overly tight. If it doesn't pass the leak test, then send it back and try another brand. Different brands fit different shapes of faces better than others.

Order a few disposable protective suits or coveralls (Tyvek® or something similar), and put a suit on before entering the house to clean. Take the suit off when you come out. One suit should last a long time. Don't worry about throwing it away unless it has holes or becomes really dirty. It's not an infectious disease we are dealing with. I suggest wearing suits because it's nice to not worry about your clothes getting dirty, and you will get dirty when you use the leaf blower.

Buy a pair of long rubber gloves, the type for washing dishes. These are better than leather work gloves and can be washed and reused.

Wear earplugs.

Full-face respirators, disposable suits, and supplies
Aramsco
(800) 767-6933
www.aramsco.com

Supplies You Will Need

Cleaning Supplies

Dish soap works best. I prefer non-fragrant soap, such as that from Seventh Generation. Get a bucket and a large bag of rags. Clean rags should not go back into the sudsy water. Other supplies may include a tall ladder and trash bags for used rags.

The intention of cleaning should be to remove spores and dust, not to treat them. Plain soap and water (what you wash dishes with) works best. Bleach does not help because it does not contain a surfactant. The chlorine ions in bleach repel from hard surfaces, making scrubbing them futile. Antimicrobials, odor bombs, and disinfectants are also wastes of effort and money.

I don't recommend vinegar, as I don't want everything to smell like vinegar. I don't like mold stain removers either, as they leave a residual film. Products that can be fogged do not remove mold. Ozone does not remove mold, and it reacts with materials and causes new odors, as do essential oils. Stick to soap and water.

A Storage or Moving Truck

Consider renting a box storage unit for temporary storage as you move things out of the house before cleaning it. This can be stored in the driveway. One

Dust Money

may rent a moving van to use for a temporary storage. This can be parked in the driveway, and one can move stuff into the van while cleaning the house.

Help

Recruit family members and friends. You may want to hire a moving crew to move stuff out of the house and into storage as well as a general cleaning crew to clean the house and its contents.

The Cleaning Process

Dust Money

Cleaning or Replacing the HVAC and its Ductwork

Have a mold inspector inspect the HVAC (heating, ventilation, and air conditioning) system and the ductwork. It can be helpful to schedule an HVAC contractor to be present during this inspection. The HVAC contractor can open access panels to make it easier for the mold inspector to look inside the system. The ASHRAE standard for inspecting and maintaining HVAC systems in commercial buildings can be used to inspect a residential system.

If the ducts got wet, ducts made with fibrous materials, such as ductboard, fiberboard, or fiberglass, should be removed and replaced with new materials. When in doubt, replace the ducts.

If the ducts and the HVAC system did not get wet, then they are only dirty and you may try to clean them. However, it can be difficult to effectively clean ducts, especially flexible ducts. Therefore, it's only practical to clean metal ducting. Flex type ducting should be replaced.

Dust Money

Duct cleaning is never 100% effective. It's not possible to clean every nook and cranny inside the ducts, furnace, and air-conditioning blower compartments. Duct cleaning is like chimney sweeping. Workers insert air hoses and brushes into each duct, and there is a fee for each duct. It adds up. To get what you pay for, you must watch the workers and make sure they spend time at each duct. Use common sense. If it seems they are going too fast to do a good job, they are.

It can be difficult to clean the blower compartment and all the components inside an HVAC system. This is a good opportunity to replace the furnace and air conditioner if they are old or on the list of upgrades. Spend the money on a new system instead of cleaning the old one. When in doubt, especially if there was a lot of mold in the house, consider replacing the HVAC system.

If you are going to have the air ducts cleaned, the ducts and the HVAC components should be cleaned prior to cleaning the house. Cleaning these components is not a mold remediator's job. Hire a duct cleaning company certified by the National Duct Cleaners Association (NADCA).

There is a standard for duct cleaning and a test for how clean the ducts are supposed to be. Both are imperfect. The testing standard is basically a white glove test. When the duct cleaning company is fin-

Cleaning the HVAC and ductwork

ished, look inside the ducts. Do a white glove test as best as possible. Look inside the system to see if the blower wheel, drip pan, and coils for the air conditioner are clean.

Want to learn more?

For inspecting furnaces, air conditioners, and ductwork, check out *ASHRAE/ACCA Standard Practice for Inspection and Maintenance of Commercial Building HVAC Systems* by the American Society of Heating, Refrigerating and Air-Conditioning Engineers, Inc. (ASHRAE) and the Air Conditioning Contractors of America (ACCA), 2008.

For air duct cleaning, check out *ACR, The NADCA Standard for Assessment, Cleaning & Restoration of HVAC Systems* by the National Air Duct Cleaners Association (NADCA), 2013.

Dust Money

Cleaning the House

Cleaning the house comes before cleaning its contents. You can't clean items inside a dirty house, and you don't want to bring items that have been cleaned into a dirty house. DO NOT clean the house until all of the following are completed:

- Any place where mold grew is dry. Mold can grow back unless repairs are made to prevent further moisture problems. Mold remediation should not have started until everything was dry. Otherwise, any mold that was removed may have grown back.

- Mold remediation is completed.

- The mold inspector inspected and tested the areas where mold remediation took place and told you that the mold (mold growth) is gone.

- You are certain there is not mold growth in the house. If you are not certain, test the suspicious areas before proceeding.

Dust Money

- If additional areas require remediation, remediate them.

- You have rebuilt any areas where mold remediation took place. Reconstruction activities generate dust from cutting, sawing, finishing drywall, and painting. It's better to clean the house after this work is completed. Whenever possible, leave the containment (plastic sheeting around the work area) in place and continue to run the air scrubber to create negative air pressure as the work area is rebuilt. Tell the mold remediation company to leave the containment up for your general contractor to use. This is a good reason to buy your own air scrubber. Mold remediators rent them for $125 per day. If you own the scrubber, you can leave it on the entire time reconstruction is taking place without worrying about how much it costs to rent.

Who to Hire to Do the Cleaning

DO NOT HIRE A PROFESSIONAL MOLD REMEDIATION COMPANY. They will not do it the way it's specified here, even if you put it in writing. You will have to supervise the workers and have an ironclad contract to enforce the methods specified. If you go that route, specify in the contract that the remedia-

Cleaning the House

tion company will not get paid until it passes post remediation testing and that the post-testing must be aggressive air testing (using a leaf blower), as specified in later chapters on testing.

Find helpers or hire a moving company to move your belongings out of the house. Then, hire a cleaning company to clean the house. At this point, the mold growth should have been removed.

The Steps

Day 1 - Pack It All Out

You must empty a house before you can clean it. Put items in boxes and move the boxes outside or into a temporary storage. You may rent a moving truck and park it in the driveway to store your belongings as you clean the house.

Inspect each item as you pack it. Throw out items that may have mold or smell like mold. If these items are keepsakes or of significant value and you want to try to restore them using advanced methods, place them in separate, designated containers to be cleaned off-site by a specialized restoration service.

Throw out or put into separate, designated containers any items that have stains from water damage, even if there is no visible mold. You may want to test

Dust Money

or inspect these more carefully.

Pack the remaining items and move them outside or into the temporary storage unit or moving van.

DAY 2 - Prepare the (Empty) House to be Cleaned

Air-handling equipment (heating, ventilation, and air conditioning) should be shut down. Supply and return vents throughout the house should be sealed with tape and plastic. If the ducts were cleaned, the air ducts and return registers should have been sealed after they were cleaned. If it's a new system, it should remain off, unused, and sealed until after the house is cleaned.

Heavy furniture and furnishings that will not be removed from the house should be wrapped and sealed with polyethylene sheeting and tape.

Carpet should be removed or covered with plastic. This is a good time to replace old carpet and padding. Carpet holds dust and is difficult to clean. In places where dust settles down to the pad, a vacuum cannot effectively remove it. If you are going to remove the carpet, remove it before using the leaf blower to clean. It's easier to vacuum a bare wood or concrete floor.

Kitchen and bathroom cabinets that will not have their interiors cleaned or are not empty, should be covered with polyethylene sheeting and sealed.

Cleaning the House

Set Up the Oscillating Fans

At least one fan should be aimed at each corner of each room. Place other fans at your discretion, aimed up walls, at the ceiling, and so forth. The purpose is to minimize stagnant air zones where dust can settle.

Set Up the Air Scrubbers

An air scrubber should be placed in the middle of each room. If you have only one scrubber, consider placing it at the center of the house. You will need at least one for each floor, or else you should clean the floors separately. Work from top to bottom.

If the scrubber was previously used (rented), it should be exhausted outdoors. Connect a plastic duct to the exhaust and run the duct outside through a window or door that is cracked. Seal around the door or window opening as best as possible with cardboard, plastic, and tape to make a tight fit around the duct. This serves to create a suction when the scrubber is running. Close the windows.

In rooms without a scrubber, consider placing box fans in windows to blow air outside.

For rooms that have neither scrubbers nor box fans, it may not be helpful to place oscillating fans, as the suspended dust will not be removed. However, you should still use the leaf blower in these rooms, followed by the vacuum, as you did for the rest of the house.

If you have enough time, take extra days to clean a few rooms each day. Place a fan and a scrubber in each room, use the leaf blower, and vacuum throughout the entire house.

Keep It Simple

It's ideal if there is an air scrubber in each room. However, this is not possible for most homeowners due to the cost of air scrubbers. When you understand the principles of cleaning stated herein, you can creatively apply them to clean an entire home with only one air scrubber.

DAY 3 - Air Wash the Interior of the House

Allocate at least one full day to this step. Turn on all the fans and air scrubbers.

Clean empty kitchen and bathroom cabinets first. Blow the insides of them with the blower, and then shut the cabinets and cover and seal them with polyethylene sheeting and tape. Do the same with the drawers. Do not proceed until all cabinets and drawers in the house are clean and sealed.

Cleaning the House

Blow

Walk through the house with a leaf blower, aiming it randomly. Direct the air stream to all corners of the rooms, ceiling, walls, tops of cabinets, steps, beams, doorjambs, light fixtures, and so forth.

Allow the Dust to Settle

Immediately after using the blower, go outside and wait for fifteen minutes. The level of airborne particles will be high. According to measurements taken with a laser particle counter, it takes approximately fifteen minutes for the dust to settle.

Vacuum

Go back inside, and HEPA vacuum the floors. The purpose of this step is to remove the bulk of the dust that blew out. It is not to perform a detailed cleaning. Don't work too hard. Just get the big stuff.

Repeat

Repeat the aforementioned steps for the duration of one full day. FOR THE CLEANING TO BE EFFECTIVE, IT IS IMPORTANT THAT THE LEAF BLOWER BE USED MULTIPLE TIMES OVER THE COURSE OF

Dust Money

A DAY WITH VACUUMING IN BETWEEN.

Move the Fans

Every two hours, reposition the fans. Moving the fans ensures that all parts of the rooms and the house get air movement and thus minimizes dead zones.

Check Your Work

When using the leaf blower does not result in hazy air or big stuff landing on the floor, the house is ready for a final cleaning. I suggest leaving the fans and air scrubbers on over night and returning in the morning to finish cleaning.

DAY 4 - Vacuum and Wipe Everything

Turn off and remove all the fans and air scrubbers from the house.

Vacuum all horizontal surfaces (floors, stairs, tops of cabinets, and so forth).

After vacuuming, use plain soap and water to damp wipe or mop all surfaces in the house. A non-fragrant dish soap is recommended. Work from top to bottom, cleaning walls, tops of cabinets, and floors. This may require a ladder to reach the upper parts of walls and

Cleaning the House

fixtures. Get a large bag of rags. Used rags should not go back into the clean water. The method to use for damp wiping is as follows: Fold a clean, sorbent rag in quarters. Dip it into the soap and water. Ring the rag to remove excess water. Apply it to a surface to be cleaned. Change the wiping surface of the rag after each pass. Used rags should not re-enter the bucket of soap and water. Used rags should be placed in plastic bags pending disposal or laundering. Rags may be laundered and reused.

Alterations to the Protocol for Cleaning the House

If you cannot use a leaf blower:

There may be instances where it's not possible or desirable to use a leaf blower. It could be that the contents are not packed out and there is a risk of breaking fragile items. This alternative is not the most effective method of cleaning, but it may result in some improvement in symptoms if the fans are numerous, repositioned during the day, and distributed throughout the house to ensure there are no stagnant air zones. This presupposes that exposure results when settled dust is disturbed.

1. Set a new air scrubber in the middle of the floor plan on each floor, placing as many oscillating fans around

Dust Money

the house as possible and setting them on high speed.

2. Leave the house for a few days, and let the fans and scrubbers run.

3. Finish by vacuuming the floor and cleaning the house with soap and water, from top to bottom.

If you can not purchase or rent an air scrubber:

An alternative plan that doesn't require an air scrubber would be to open all the windows. Note that this method of cleaning may be much less effective. Most of the dust will settle out quickly after using the leaf blower. If you don't have an air scrubber, you may want to skip using oscillating fans and reduce the entire cleaning procedure to using a leaf blower followed by HEPA vacuuming. Finish by cleaning with soap and water from top to bottom.

Cleaning an entire house with one air scrubber:

PART 1

The house should have been prepped as previously explained: seal cabinets that won't be cleaned, shut off and seal the HVAC system, seal air supply and return air ducts.

Clean the top floor first. Place the air scrubber in the

Cleaning the House

first room. Do not worry about using oscillating fans.

Walk through the house (floor) with the leaf blower. Blow all the rooms with the leaf blower, including both the room with the scrubber and those without. Go outside, and wait fifteen minutes.

Go inside. Vacuum the floors in ALL the rooms in the house.

Move the scrubber to the next room. Close the door to the room that was cleaned.

Repeat for all other rooms in the house: walk through the house (floor) with the leaf blower, and blow ALL the rooms. Go outside and wait fifteen minutes. Come back inside, and vacuum the floors in ALL the rooms.

Move the scrubber to the next room, seal the room that last contained the air scrubber, and continue until all the rooms have had a turn.

Remember to change the pre-filters on the air scrubber as they become dirty. You should have ordered a case of each pre-filter. Don't be shy about using them. If the pre-filters become clogged, air bypasses them, causing the HEPA filter (an expensive filter) to become dirtier and shortening its life. Some use duct tape to seal around the edges of the pre-filters where they are installed in the scrubber to prevent air from bypassing them.

Dust Money

PART 2

Move the air scrubber to the middle of the floor plan.

Place the oscillating fans in each room, and turn them on. There should be fans in each room to keep dust particles suspended. Ideally, one fan should be aimed at each corner of each room. Other fans may be aimed, at discretion, up the walls, at the ceiling, and so forth.

Once all the fans and the air scrubber are running, leave them for an entire day, occasionally coming inside to move the fans around so they randomly hit other corners and places to minimize stagnant zones.

Leave the fans and the scrubber on overnight.

In the morning, turn everything off.

Vacuum all the floors in each room. If there are lower floors to be cleaned, vacuum the lower floors too.

PART 3

You should have started with the top floor. Move the equipment to the lower floor. (If you have only one floor, skip to Part 4). If possible, seal the entry to the upper floor with plastic. Repeat Part 2 for the lower floors.

Cleaning the House

PART 4

This is the final step of cleaning and requires the most elbow grease. Open the windows. (The windows should have been closed while the scrubbers were running to make them more effective). Remove the fans and air scrubbers from the building.

Vacuum all surfaces from top to bottom as best as possible, including the ceiling, the walls, and then the floor. If your vacuum is not a HEPA vacuum (highly recommended), consider turning the air scrubber on and moving it with you as you go to clear the air so you don't breathe the dust that blows out of the vacuum.

After vacuuming, damp wipe or mop all surfaces from top to bottom, including the ceiling, the walls, and then the floors.

Should You Test the House?

If you followed the cleaning protocol and all the actual mold growth was removed before you started, you should not need any testing. Testing is covered in later chapters for those who are interested. It can take several days to receive testing results. If you choose to have testing done, the house should remain empty until the results are back from the laboratory and indicate that the house is clean. You will need a mold

Dust Money

inspector with a vacuum pump and a flow meter to do the testing. If you hire an inspector, make sure that they are a CMC (Certified Microbial Consultant) with a certification from ACAC.ORG (American Council for Accredited Certification). Testing will cost a minimum of several hundred to a thousand dollars, depending on how big your house is and how confident you want to be in the results.

Cleaning Contents (Belongings)

It's difficult to say how critical it is to clean the contents of a house that had mold. It depends on how moldy the house was and how sensitive the occupants are. This assumes that any contents that had visible mold were discarded. Sensitive people can be bothered by only a few spores in the dust, while others don't appear to be bothered. You may choose to be more or less thorough, depending on your level of concern. If you are moving, you may choose to dust and clean items as you would normally when moving. If you are sensitive, immunocompromised, or for reasons wish to clean the contents of the house as best as possible, follow the following protocol to the letter.

There's no sense in cleaning the contents if the house is dirty. Proceed only after the house has been cleaned. Items should have been packed into boxes and moved to storage as the house was cleaned.

If you're not sure or don't want to put in the effort to clean a particular item, consider disposing of it. If

Dust Money

you're not sure whether you want to get rid of something, cover and seal the item with plastic and store it while you clean the remainder of the items.

This is a big job. Get family members and friends to help. Most people short cut this process and do the best they can. Be prepared to have patience. You can't see the spores you are cleaning.

Throw the Bad Stuff Away

Separate items that got wet and have visible mold from those that were simply in the same room where mold was growing. If you see mold on an item, or if an item smells like mold, throw it away.

Clean the Rest

If something did not get wet, mold cannot grow on it. Clean such items as you would normally clean something that is dusty. In the following steps, you're going to use a leaf blower or compressed air hose to blow dust off of them, vacuum them as best as possible, and wipe or wash them with plain soap and water. You can launder cloths with regular laundry soap. Take porous items like couches or bedding outdoors and beat them with a stick (while wearing a respirator). Do not bother using bleach, chemicals, or biocides. They are not going to help and may create new, objectionable odors or may be irritating.

Cleaning Contents (Belongings)

Gather Spring Cleaning Tools

- Bucket of water and fragrance-free dish soap
- Large bag of rags
- Vacuum cleaner
- Leaf blower
- Compressed air hose (optional)

Organize Items into Groups Based on Types of Material

- Porous items (books, cloths, and bedding)
- Semi-porous items (wood furniture)
- Non-porous items (metal and glass)

The Procedure for Cleaning Belongings (Contents of the House)

Clean items outside.

Anything that can be washed should be washed. Washing is more effective than vacuuming or wiping. Have two washtubs: one with soapy water and another for rinsing. It may be helpful to have folding tables set up on which to place washed items to dry. These should be placed down wind, and away from the cleaning area, where the leaf blower or compressed air hose is being used. A second moving van may be helpful to move clean items into in the event that you can

Dust Money

not immediately move them into the house. Moving items into the garage is OK if the garage was cleaned when the house was cleaned.

Hard items (e.g., plastic, metal, wood, and glass) are easy to clean. Wipe these down with soap and water or wash them. An example is a wood dining table with a glass tabletop. Simply wipe the top, legs, and bottom with rags dipped in soap and water. The rags should be damp, not wet. The items should not become so visibly wet that they require a significant amount of time to dry. After cleaning the items, move them to a location where they are not exposed to dust blown into the air by the leaf blower or compressed air hose. Move them into the (clean) house or a second storage van for temporary storage. (The first storage van will contain dirty items).

Cloths are easy to clean. Use regular laundry soap. Use fragrance-free laundry soap, as the fragrance in laundry soap is known to aggravate allergy symptoms.

Use a compressed air house to clean the nooks and crannies of items for which a vacuum cleaner or damp wipe would not be effective. A computer is an example of an item that would benefit from the leaf blower or compressed air hose. The compressed air hose or leaf blower should be used with caution, as things can break if. they are blown too hard. Wear a full-face or half-face respirator, goggles for eye protection, and ear plugs.

Cleaning Contents (Belongings)

The sequence to clean items is as follows:

1. **Wash it with soapy water.** If an item can tolerate being submerged, wash the item in soap and water. Consider using the dishwasher to wash small items. If you are able to wash an item, move it to a clean location where it can dry, such as a garage or a second moving van i.e., a place where it will not be dirtied by dust from outside or from the cleaning station. If you wash an item, skip the remaining steps. Washing will clean it as best as possible.

2. **Air-wash it**. For items that cannot be washed by submerging them in soapy water, this is the most important and effective step. Blow items with a compressed air hose or leaf blower. This works particularly well for items such as books. One way is to put a stack of books in a box, aim the leaf blower into it (wearing goggles or a full-face respirator), and randomly flip pages and agitate the books. Another would be to clean one book at a time, flipping the pages and hitting the tops and sides. Afterward, pack the books into a clean box or move them into the house.

The leaf blower works especially well for boxes of small knickknacks. Place items in a clean, small-to-medium-sized box. Aim the blower into the box, taking care not to break or otherwise damage fragile items. Move the items around as you hit them with a stream of air. When you are finished, move them into

Dust Money

the house or to a clean storage location.

3. **Vacuum it.** You may use any type of vacuum. A HEPA vacuum is not required, as this activity is performed outside. Although using a blower or compressed air hose is generally more effective than vacuuming, vacuuming is appropriate for some items. I will use an upholstered couch as an example. First, I would use the blower on it after removing the cushions. Then, I'd beat the cushions outside with a big stick. (All the cleaning of the household contents should be done outside). Finally, I'd vacuum the cushions and couch for good measure. That's the best you can do for this type of item. If you can't remove the dust (i.e., mold spores in the settled dust) from the piece through these activities, you are not going to disturb and aerosolize enough spores such that an exposure results when you sit on the couch.

4. **Wipe it.** The last step in the cleaning process is damp wiping. If it can't be washed, damp wipe it with soap and water as best as possible after using the leaf blower or compressed air hose to blow the dust off of.

Testing

Testing a House

You will need a mold inspector to do testing. Most mold inspectors charge $100 per air sample in addition to their fee, which can average $500 or more. You could do testing yourself, but you would need equipment and an understanding of how to use it, which is beyond the scope of this book. I will provide a brief overview of how this equipment works and how testing is performed. The house should remain empty until test results are returned from the laboratory, which may take several days. Do not bring any belongings back into the house until you receive results that indicate that the house is clean.

How It's Done

A vacuum pump, a flow meter to calibrate the pump, and spore trap cassettes for air samples are required for testing. The pump is used to pull air into the sample cassettes. In order for the test to be meaningful,

Dust Money

you need to know how much air is collected and compare that value to that of a baseline sample collected before the leaf blower is used to disturb the dust in the home.

Inside the sample cassette is a sticky, glass microscope slide. As air is pulled into it, particles (e.g., mold, dust, insulation, skin cells, and pollen) stick to the slide. Air samples are typically collected for 5 to 10 minutes each. Then, these samples are sent to a laboratory, where the analyst removes the slide from the cassette and looks at it under a microscope. He or she looks for mold spores (there will always be some) and counts them. The result is a count of each type of spore present per the volume of air collected, spores per liter of air.

Twenty-four hours before testing is to be done, close the windows (if they were open) and turn off and remove the air scrubbers. Turn off the heating or air conditioning system, and cover the air supply and return air vents. (The HVAC system should have been left off and sealed after the system and ducts were cleaned).

Next, you will mimic what happens when the settled dust is disturbed. This is done by taking samples indoors before and after using the leaf blower. I suggest you have the mold inspector collect two air samples indoors in the middle of the floor plan with all the doors open between rooms. These samples should

Testing

be collected in the same spot. Average the results, and treat them as one sample. If there is more than one floor, collect two samples on each floor in the middle of the floor plan. This is the minimum number of tests. You may collect more. Always collect a minimum of two samples in each location.

After collecting the air samples under normal conditions, put on PPE (a full-face HEPA filter respirator and ear plugs). The contents should have been packed out so that nothing is damaged or dirty. Wave the blower around as you walk through the house. Wave it at the tops of door jambs and light fixtures. Take care, as needed, not to wave the leaf blower directly at any remaining contents or parts of the structure that could be damaged. This should take less than five minutes. Next, go outside and wait for the dust to settle. Waiting allows the big stuff to settle out of the air. If this is not done, the air samples will be overloaded with background dust and the laboratory won't be able to see any mold spores for all the dust.

While waiting for the dust to settle, take at least one outdoor air sample. It can be collected anywhere outside, such as a patio, the driveway, or a porch.

Go back inside, and collect a second set of air samples from the same locations. Do not collect these for the same amount of time as for the first set. There will still be a lot of particles in the air. Take these for approximately two minutes each, depending on how dusty the house is. Ask your mold inspector to hold the cassette up to the light to check the amount of background debris on the slide. If he can't see through the slide for all the dust, collect the samples over for a shorter amount of time. The house may be dirtier than it appears.

Send the samples to a laboratory, noting the amount of time over which each sample was collected. You can now open the doors and windows. If there are air scrubbers, turn them on to help flush the air.

Interpreting Laboratory Results

The total concentrations of mold spores detected in the air indoors after a blower is used will be higher than those under normal conditions both outside and inside under normal conditions. Comparing the level of spores indoors to that outdoors is not logical. If you do so, the house will appear to be dirty and contaminated with mold. A determination as to whether mold contamination exists is made by comparing the types of mold detected in air samples before and after a blower is used. The relative percentages of each type should be similar. *Cladosporium* is the genus that is most predominantly isolated both indoors and outdoors, followed by basidiospores (mushrooms and rot spores), *Aspergillus/Penicillium*-like spores, and

Testing

Alternaria.

A problem interior may be one in which *Aspergillus/Penicillium*-like spores are the dominant genera (greater than 50%). That, however, is not a hard rule, as *Aspergillus/Penicillium*-like spores may consist of *Aspergillus, Penicillium,* or one of numerous other molds that have clear, round, and small spores chained together like beads on a pearl necklace. A less-than-desirable level of *Aspergillus/Penicillium*-like spores does not automatically mean contamination is present.

Chaetomium, Fusarium, and *Stachybotrys* are indicator molds. The detection of a few spores of any of these is significant and may indicate contamination, either in the settled dust or in mold hiding in the walls or ceiling. The source of contamination cannot be determined by collecting air samples. If you are certain that there is nowhere in the house where mold growth could be hiding, then it is possible that the house has not been cleaned adequately. If, however, there is some doubt as to whether mold growth could be hiding somewhere, then the mold inspector should be called back to do more testing for hidden mold.

DID YOU KNOW?

Some mistakenly call *Stachybotrys* a species of mold. *Stachybotrys* is a genus. A common species of *Stachybotrys* is *Stachybotrys chatarum.*

Dust Money

In the following example, you can see that after using a leaf blower, the number of spores detected for each type of mold went up proportionally. The exception was *Stachybotrys*, which was not detected before the blower was used. This suggests that the house is dirty, as spores of *Stachybotrys* are in the settled dust. Another was the level of *Aspergillus/Penicillium*. It skyrocketed after the blower was used.

Spore Counts / m³	Air in the House	
	Normal, Quiet (Before Blower)	Disturbed (After Blower)
Alternaria	4	67
Ascospores	27	67
Basidiospores	67	130
Chaetomium	7	130
Cladosporium	120	600
Aspergillus/Penicillium types	205	160,000
Stachybotrys		930
Total Spores (Counts / m³)	485	160,000

Testing Household Contents (Belongings)

It's not generally recommended to test household contents and belongings. Logically, if there was mold in a house, items were in the house, and the surfaces of those items were exposed to dust settling, then the

Testing

items should be contaminated with settled spores. It's not a question of if but how much. If could be negligible (hard to detect) or significant (capable of causing a reaction in those who would otherwise not consider themselves sensitive). Because of the variation of individual susceptibility, it is not possible to determine a safe level of settled spores. The general recommendation is to clean items instead of testing them.

It is time-consuming and expensive to test individual items. If something looks or smells moldy, throw it out. If something got wet and didn't dry fast enough, consider throwing it out. If there is an insurance claim on certain items, save those items in case the adjuster wants to inventory or salvage them.

How It's Done

The procedure for testing contents and belongings is similar to that for testing a house. It requires the proper equipment and an understanding of how to use this equipment as previously explained.

STEP 1

Find a clean space into which you can move the items that you want to test. This can be a storage unit or a moving van. Clean the space using a leaf blower, a vacuum, and soap and water.

Dust Money

STEP 2

Before moving the contents into the storage space or van, test the space to make sure that it's clean. The door to the space should be kept closed for 24 hours before testing. As with testing the house, collect two indoor air samples and at least one outdoor sample as a reference. After collecting indoor samples under normal conditions, turn on the leaf blower and wave it around inside for a few moments. Next, go outside, wait fifteen minutes, go back inside, take another set of air samples, and then send them to the laboratory. Compare the results of the samples collected before using the blower to those collected after using the blower. Follow the aforementioned guidelines to interpret the laboratory results. If the space appears questionable or dirty, find a different location for testing. If, based on the test results, the space appears to be clean, proceed to move contents and belongings into it for testing.

STEP 3

Move the contents (belongings) into the clean storage space. Typically, this involves moving boxes of contents. There are creative ways to do this. For example, you could set up folding tables inside the space, unpack the contents, and spread them out on the

Testing

tables or simply open the boxes once they have been moved into the space.

Collect two air samples in the space under normal conditions. Then, use a leaf blower to blow the dust off of the contents. Keep the door to the storage or moving van closed to limit the amount of outdoor air that enters it. If the contents are still in boxes, open the boxes and hit the contents with a stream of air. After blowing the contents with the leaf blower, go outside and wait ten minutes for the dust to settle. Then, go back inside to collect two air samples, collect an outdoor sample, and send the samples to a laboratory. When you get the results, look for species that don't belong. These are *Stachybotrys* and *Chaetomium*.

The difficult part is determining what to do if the results fail the criteria required to confirm that the contents are clean. Since you won't be testing every item, you won't know which ones are more or less contaminated. If the test suggests the items are contaminated, you will have to reclean everything. This is not likely to happen if 1) you throw out items that are wet, appear moldy, or smell moldy as you are packing; 2) you rigorously follow the cleaning protocol.

Dust Money

The Environmental Relative Mold Index (ERMI)

What is It?

In the early 2000s, a realtor told me that I didn't know what I was doing because I wasn't using the Relative Moldiness Index (RMI), what would later become the Environmental Relative Mold Index (ERMI). I quietly accepted the criticism. I had never heard of the test. They didn't teach us about it in the courses I took to study for my certification as a mold inspector.

A short time later, I attended a conference at which the Environmental Protection Agency (EPA) presented on the test. It was not being developed as a better test for professionals to use. Rather, the purpose was to find a cheaper and easier way for homeowners to test for mold.

To use the ERMI, a homeowner must collect a sample of dust from their home using a dust swifter or vacuum. Then, the laboratory tests the dust sample for

Dust Money

spores and fragments of various species of molds using a type of DNA test. The results are compared to what is considered to be a normal amount of mold burden for a home.

Concerns

When the presenters finished, I raised my hand to ask questions. First, I asked from which cities were the samples collected to establish what level of mold is considered normal. You can't get a house in Arizona as clean as one in Florida. There's more outdoor mold spores in climates like Florida, which settle in the dust inside.

The presenters would not answer the question. At the time, I didn't understand the secrecy. Later, I discovered that the scientists receive a percentage of the royalties paid to the EPA from laboratories that analyze samples. I noticed this while reading the paper "Development of an Environmental Relative Moldiness Index for US Homes" in the fine print under the abstract. I had to wait until 2008 to get an answer: Ohio. The EPA's office was located in Cincinnati. Meanwhile, under heavy marketing from laboratories, homeowners, mold remediators, and home inspectors started using the ERMI.

My next question was for the other professionals in the room, my colleagues. I asked for a show of hands

The ERMI Test

from anyone who had used the ERMI and found that if they had not, they would have made an error and failed to detect mold in a home. No one raised their hand.

Level of *Stachybotrys* Detected	
ERMI Test	**Air Sample**
29 E/mg (spore equivalents per milligram of dust)	15 spores 500 spores per liter of air 130 hyphal fragments

Comparison of ERMI results, for which the homeowner collected a dust sample, to the results of an air sample that I collected after I had turned on an oscillating fan in the living room. Both the ERMI and the air sample detected Stachybotrys. The air sample cost less.

Time Marches On

The EPA realized that it needed to expand the number of cites from which it collected samples if the ERMI was to be representative of mold levels outside of Ohio. In 2006, working with the Department of Housing and Urban Development (HUD), they expanded the number of cities from which dust samples were collected. The names of these cities have not

Dust Money

been disclosed. Based on a 2008 article published in the Journal of Occupational and Environmental Medicine, we can speculate. The collection of additional samples for the ERMI study was piggy-backed on a national survey to study levels of lead-based paint in homes as part of the HUD's American Healthy Home Survey.

A homeowner using the ERMI may expect that the sample collected from their home will be compared to average homes across America. Not quite. The homes tested were HUD Section 8 units, which are in a program through which the government provides assistance to landlords on behalf of low-income tenants. A housing unit was defined as a house, apartment, mobile home, group of homes, or single room occu-

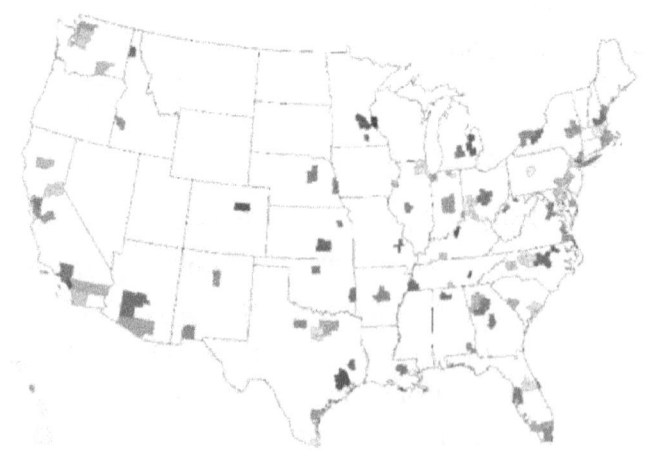

Locations surveyed in the 2008 AHHA study.

The ERMI Test

pied as a separate living quarters. Of those selected to participate, only 1,131 tenants completed the survey. If you use the ERMI, your results will be compared against those 1,131 units.

How the ERMI Can Be Improved

A study in Finland determined the applicability of the ERMI to Finnish residences. Researchers found an agreement between the ERMI and visible mold but only in houses with severe manifestations of visible mold. The researches tweaked the ERMI and created the FERMI, which was found to be a good predictor of mold for the climate and types of mold found in Finland. The study also revealed significantly higher ERMI values in the winter, which were explained by a reduction in the number of outdoor spores that settle indoors during the winter. Higher ERMI values were obtained in the winter when doors and windows were closed.

One thing I didn't ask the EPA about was how they decided which species to test for. The ERMI is a DNA test. It's expensive to do, and 70,000 species of mold are estimated to exist. Each species would need to be tested for separately. To reduce the cost, the EPA tests for a reduced number of species. Molds with the highest national average concentrations were selected to be included. The ERMI may, therefore, be thought of as

Dust Money

a relative index to the most common types of mold found outdoors across the United States, which is not useful for determining whether there is mold in your home.

I have additional concerns about the ERMI. Mold spores have thick outer shells made of chitin, one of the hardest known substances. The ERMI cannot detect DNA inside a spore. The laboratory must break the spores open. They do this by grinding the dust sample with a metal roller like that used by a baker to roll dough.

Much of the processes, equipment, and chemicals used by laboratories to analyze ERMI samples have not been validated or disclosed. I didn't realize, for example, that ERMI results could be skewed by chemicals present in house dust until a client sent me an ERMI report in which the laboratory had hand written the following comment:

> *"Results are skewed due to chemical found in dust sample -- chemical interferes w/ test results. (Our lab) can't say whether the mold results should be higher or lower than what's reported... just that the #'s are skewed."*

After the ERMI was introduced, mold remediators started using it to convince homeowners that remediation was necessary. Homeowners have failed to ask on what level of the ERMI scale their house should be

The ERMI Test

to conclude the mold was gone (or that there wasn't any to begin with). After spending tens of thousands of dollars but failing to achieve the low ERMI scores they desired, people complained to the Office of the Inspector General (OIG). In 2013, the OIG required the EPA to release a statement reminding people that the ERMI is a research project and not intended for public use. They substantiated allegations that many of the homes tested did not need mold remediation.

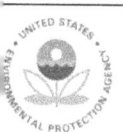

U.S. Environmental Protection Agency
Office of Inspector General

13-P-0356
August 22, 2013

At a Glance

Why We Did This Review

An Office of Inspector General hotline complaint alleged that firms were using the U.S. Environmental Protection Agency-developed Environmental Relative Moldiness Index tool to evaluate homes for indoor mold even though the EPA had not validated the tool for public use. The EPA developed ERMI as a

Public May Be Making Indoor Mold Cleanup Decisions Based on EPA Tool Developed Only for Research Applications

What We Found

We substantiated the allegation that firms were using the mold index tool although the EPA had not validated the tool for public use. The EPA readily acknowledged that it had not validated or peer reviewed MSQPCR or ERMI for public use. The agency said it considers MSQPCR and ERMI to be research tools not intended for public use. Although the EPA has licensed MSQPCR to companies for introduction into the marketplace under the Federal Technology Transfer Act of 1986, neither federal law nor the EPA's procedures address the level of validation needed before or after transferring federally developed

Doctor Knows Best?

Some doctors recommend the ERMI to their patients as a method of testing a home to see if there is mold in it. Doctors like the ERMI because they say traditional air samples do not detect mold. However, this assertion is

Dust Money

taken out of context.

When doctors say "air samples," they are referring to what is commonly done when a homeowner asks a mold inspector to do a mold test. The air samples collected are called spore traps and consist of sticky glass slides onto which airborne particles stick. Spore traps have become the normal way of collecting air samples because they are easy to collect and have a fast turnaround time. Doctors are correct in saying that a single spore trap may not detect mold growing in a home. However, they are incorrect in saying that air samples do not detect mold growth in a home.

Prior to the mid 2000s, we collected several different types of air samples; this is a good way of using air samples to test for mold. We collected spore traps as well as second and third sets of cultured air samples. Doing so tripled the cost of testing, and it took as long as ten days to receive results from the laboratory. As more home inspectors became "mold inspectors," they were trained to keep things simple and price competitive. They were also trained to collect spore traps. Many have never heard of culturing air samples. An Anderson sampler is required to collect cultured air samples, and cannot be found in most mold inspector's tool boxes.

Just as a doctor must choose a type of media to culture a swab taken from a nose or throat, so must a mold inspector choose which types of agar to use to

The ERMI Test

collect air samples for a culture. As it turns out, not all molds like the same type of food. Some grow better and faster in different types of agars. To get accurate air sampling results, it's best to use two or three types of agar: malt or potato dextrose agar for general types of fungi; a cellulose-rich agar high in water content for molds such as *Stachybotrys;* and a third agar for actinomycetes, a group of gram-positive bacteria associated with damp soil. Doing this involves collecting a dozen or more air samples. The complexity and cost of this sampling strategy is one reason for which the EPA decided to attempt to invent an alternative method to test for mold, such as the ERMI.

Those who are critical of using air samples to detect mold in a home are correct if they refer to using only one or two air samples. However, they are incorrect to say that air samples do not detect mold. Your chances of determining whether there a mold in the house can be as high as 90% if you test the air using both spore traps and a variety of agar plates (using an Anderson sampler). If you test using only spore traps, this chance may only be 50%.

Making Better Use of the ERMI

Consider the following in order to increase the accuracy of the results and make better decisions. I don't recommend using the ERMI as a method of checking

Dust Money

whether a house or its contents are contaminated with settled spores. Test the contents as discussed in previous chapters.

1. Test in the spring or summer. Do not test in the winter when doors and windows are closed.

2. Collect two samples indoors. This allows for a buddy check. The results should be similar. If they are not, then retest.

3. Collect two samples outside. Use this as a baseline to compare the types and levels of mold detected indoors to those detected outside. If you think you have a mold problem inside because a certain type of mold was detected but this mold was also detected outside, chances are it came from outside.

4. Make sure the dust you collect inside is as old as the dust collected outside. Don't collect dust indoors from a counter top that was cleaned last week and then collect dust outside from the top of a light fixture that has never been cleaned. One way to do this is to clean a surface indoors (e.g., the top of a book shelf or glass table) and a surface outside (e.g., the top of a glass patio table). Allow dust to settle on each for a minimum of two weeks before collecting dust samples. Remember to collect two samples from each. That's right—divide the glass table or counter top in half, and collect one sample from each side. If there truly is

The ERMI Test

mold, then the results should look similar. If one sample appears to be high in mold and the other appears normal, what's happened is likely that one sample had a blob of dust with mold land on it. It may not be representative of the dust in the house. The two sample results should look similar before you use them to determine whether your home is contaminated with mold. If they look dissimilar, retest.

After one client of mine received a high ERMI result, I suggested they test again with two indoor samples. The molds of concern, *Stachybotrys* and *Wallemia*, showed up in both. That piqued my interest. I had inspected and tested the house using methods other than the ERMI and had not found any mold. I suggested the client collect dust from outside and send it to the lab for an ERMI. The results of the outdoor ERMI

	Spore E./mg
Fungal ID \ Sample ID	**C12569/HC**
Aspergillus penicillioides	4
Aspergillus versicolor	ND
Chaetomium globosum	ND
Stachybotrys chartarum	2
Wallemia sebi	5

ERMI results for a sample of dust collected outside. Low levels of Stachybotrys and Wallemia (near detection limits) were detected.

Dust Money

detected *Stachybotrys* and *Wallemia*.

I returned to the house to look for an outdoor source. I didn't see any moldy grass nearby. It was a rural neighborhood. These are DNA tests. If you look for a needle in a haystack, you may find one. That doesn't mean the source is in your house.

To make better use of ERMI tests, consider the following when you receive the results:

- *Stachybotrys* does not belong indoors. If it's detected in both indoor dust samples at levels significantly higher than the detection limits, then there may be mold growing indoors or remaining in the dust from remediation activities (this is the reason for which cleaning is so important). The location of the mold cannot be determined using the ERMI.
- Don't be alarmed by small numbers. Avoid jumping to conclusions when the number reported is close to the detection limits.
- Make sure that the molds of concern are present in both indoor samples and in similar amounts.
- Take an outdoor ERMI (or two), and make sure that the molds of concern that were detected indoors were not detected outside.
- Many homeowners panic when they see that *Stachybotrys* was detected. Consider that *Stachybotrys* was detected in 38% of the samples

The ERMI Test

on which the ERMI is based. Before you worry, consider that *Stachybotrys* should be detected in both indoor samples at levels higher than the detection limit.

When the EPA began developing the ERMI, the intention was to develop a simple, cost-effective test that any homeowner could use. Considering that the average cost of the ERMI is $300 per sample and that you need at least three samples to be confident in the results, things didn't work out as planned. You can get a professional mold inspection with testing for that price. With an inspection, you'll also have some idea as to where to look for the mold. The ERMI does not tell you where the mold is or whether it came from outside or from mold in your house.

"Development of an Environmental Relative Moldiness Index for US Homes." Journal of Occupational and Environmental Medicine. August 2007, Volume 49, Issue 8, pp. 829—833.

"Public May Be Making Indoor Mold Cleanup Decisions Based on EPA Tool Developed Only for Research Applications." U.S. Environmental Protection Agency, Office of the Inspector General. 13-P-0356. August 22, 2013.

Dust Money

"Application of the Environmental Relative Moldiness Index in Finland." Applied and Environmental Microbiology. 2016 Jan 15; 82(2): 578–584.

"Quantitative PCR analysis of fungi in dust from homes of infants who developed idiopathic pulmonary hemorrhaging." Vesper SJ, Varma M, Wymer LJ, Dearborn DG, Sobolewski J, Haugland RA. Journal of Occupational and Environmental Medicine. 2004; 46:596–601.

"Quantitative PCR analysis of house dust can reveal abnormal mold conditions". Meklin T, Haugland RA, Reponen T, et al. Journal of Occupational and Environmental Medicine. 2004; 6:615–20.

Final Words

If you're reading this book, you may be experiencing intense feelings of frustration and helplessness with regard to why you are not feeling good in your home after a mold remediation project. If you are certain that the mold was removed, then what you are likely reacting to is what's left in the dust in the house.

Some think the answer is to fog the house with a product that claims to neutralize or get rid of mold. These includes products that have hydrogen peroxide, enzymes, citrus-based solutions, and so forth. Nothing of the sort will help you clean your house. Consider, can you clean (remove) normal house dust by fogging? No, you cannot. There is no such magic product.

The good news is that you can make an improvement simply by cleaning the house. Treat it as a spring cleaning project. Use a leaf blower (after you pack your stuff out). Use an air scrubber. This provides the best system for cleaning a house. I know this is a lot of work, and wish I could tell you there is

Dust Money

an easier way. It is worth it. But you can't take short cuts.

Before you clean the house, be sure that you and a mold inspector do testing and identify all the places mold is growing, as I explained in *Mold Money - How to Save Thousands of Dollars on Mold Remediation and Make Sure the Mold is Gone*. Hire a contractor or mold remediation company to remove it. Make sure that they remove (not only treat) the mold that was growing. Then, with help, clean the house and your belongings.

I wish you well.

About the Author

Daniel Stih is an aerospace engineer and consultant who investigates homes and offices to solve complaints and health problems related to being indoors. He got started after retiring as an engineer and working as a handyman. He discovered that some of his clients who were sick had things wrong with the buildings they lived in, making it difficult for them to become well again. He began to find ways of testing for and removing these issues so they could feel well again.

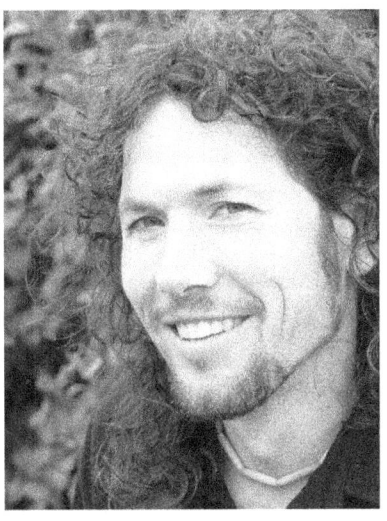
Photo by John Mate

Visit healthylivingspaces.com

Dust Money

Standards

ANSI/IICRC S520 Standard (and Reference Guide) for Professional Mold Remediation, Institute of Inspection, Cleaning and Restoration Certification (IICRC)

This is the only professional standard for mold remediation. This document has been through a tedious public review process. It is the only standard that covers evaluating and cleaning contents (belongings) and cross-contamination. The text contains definitions that differentiate between actual mold growth, cross-contamination, and normal (outside) fungal ecologies. It costs $125.

Dust Money

Guidelines

GUIDELINES ON ASSESSMENT AND REMEDIATION OF FUNGI IN INDOOR ENVIRONMENTS BY THE NEW YORK CITY DEPARTMENT OF HEALTH

This was the first public document to be published on mold remediation. These guidelines are generally good, with the exception regarding the recommendations based on the square feet of visible mold present. Most remediators would be out of a job if they based estimates on the amount of mold visible. Most of the time, most of the mold is hidden inside walls and remains hidden until the walls are cut open. Many, including some insurance companies, reference the square foot guidelines without knowing how they were created. (That's a story for another book. It'd be a short story. The square foot guidelines are not based on studies rather, they were based on the most the person assigned to write the guidelines could do at the time: a guess). The good thing about these guidelines is the emphasis on removing rather than treating mold. These guidelines say to use soap and water, to use "the gentlest detergent possible", and not to use bleach. Further, this document is a free publication and can be downloaded.

Dust Money

MOLD REMEDIATION IN SCHOOLS AND COMMERCIAL BUILDINGS (MARCH 2001) BY THE UNITED STATES ENVIRONMENTAL PROTECTION AGENCY (EPA)

A BRIEF GUIDE TO MOLD, MOISTURE AND YOUR HOME (2002) BY THE UNITED STATES ENVIRONMENTAL PROTECTION AGENCY (EPA)

I don't reference the EPA guidelines because they were copied verbatim from New York's guidelines, and unlike New York, the EPA has not updated their guidelines. Along these lines, Florida's mold laws were copied verbatim from the EPA's guidelines.

References

DAMP INDOOR SPACES AND HEALTH BY THE INSTITUTE OF MEDICINE OF THE NATIONAL ACADEMIES, THE NATIONAL ACADEMIES PRESS, WASHINGTON, D.C., 2004.

I like this book because it discusses the health effects of things that grow in buildings other than mold. This text is available online for public viewing if you don't want to buy a hardcover.
http://books.nap.edu/openbook.php?record_id=11011

HOW TO DETERMINE AND SUCCESSFULLY CLEAN UP CONDITION 2 SETTLED SPORES - AN UPDATE, BY WILLIAM VAUGHAN, PHD, QEP, CIEC, PRESENTED AT THE 13TH ANNUAL INDOOR AIR QUALITY ASSOCIATION (IAQA) MEETING, AUSTIN, TX, 2010.

This is a technical paper not intended for the layperson. You may recommend it to your mold inspector. It discusses the process and concepts of using a leaf blower to disturb the dust in a home to test for settled spores and cross-contamination, as well as the cleaning protocol to follow this process.

Dust Money

www.ingramcontent.com/pod-product-compliance
Lightning Source LLC
Chambersburg PA
CBHW070545170426
43200CB00011B/2560